THE VEGAN FITNESS

COOKBOOK

An Ultimate Step-By-Step Guide To Speeding-Up Your Fat Loss, Muscles Growth And Become A Fitness Freak In Less Than 30 Days Including 50+ Mouth-Watering And Pure Vegetarian Recipes.

BY

Sophia Moore

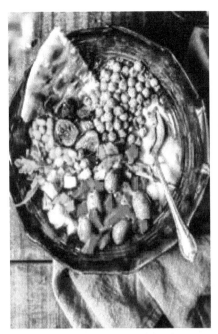

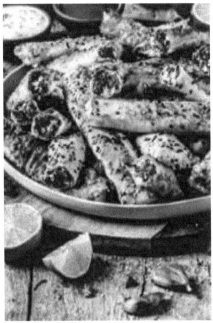

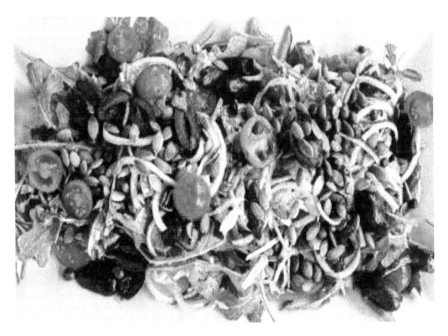

Table of Contents

INTRODUCTION

You can get all the supplements you need from a sound, adjusted vegan diet rich in wholefoods including natural products, vegetables, beats, grains, nuts, and seeds. A few investigations have revealed that individuals who eat vegan will in general burn-through more fiber, cell reinforcements, potassium, magnesium, folate, and nutrients A, C, and E.

 Eating vegan lessens our danger of experiencing malignancy and different sicknesses.

A new report proposes that eating vegan can help diminish our danger for sickness, as plant-based food sources are loaded with phytochemicals – including the amazing cell reinforcements found in products of the soil. Scientists found that vegans had higher groupings of cancer prevention agent carotenoids, a higher extent of complete omega-3 unsaturated fats, and lower levels of immersed unsaturated fats than non-vegans, all of which are connected to positive wellbeing results.

A 11-year German investigation including in excess of 800 vegan men likewise found that their malignant growth rates were not exactly a large portion of those of the overall population.

It's a given that after a humane way of life that tries not to hurt creatures will give you a more clear inner voice, and studies show that vegans may actually be more joyful than meat-eaters. Truth be told, vegans and veggie lovers would be advised to scores on gloom tests and disposition profiles than the individuals who ate fish and meat.

Most vegan food varieties contain altogether less soaked fat than creature "items" do, and numerous investigations have shown that vegans will in general have lower weight files than non-vegans.

1. Vegan Chipotle Lentil Tacos

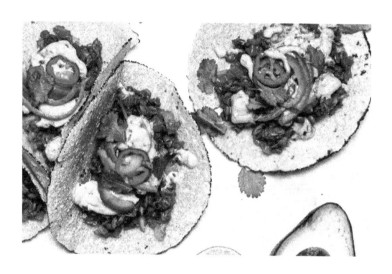

YIELDS:34 SERVINGSPREP
TIME:0 HOURS 15 MINSTOTAL
TIME:0 HOURS 40 MINS

INGREDIENTS:

- FOR LENTIL FILLING:
- 2 1/2 c. cooked green lentils (from around 1 cup dried)
- 1 tbsp. extra-virgin olive oil
- 1/2 yellow onion, finely chopped
- 2 garlic cloves, minced
- 3 tbsp. tomato paste
- 1 chipotle pepper in adobo sauce
- 1 tsp. ground cumin
- 1/2 tsp. ground coriander

- Genuine salt
- FOR CREAMY AVOCADO SAUCE:
- 1/2 avocado
- Juice of 1 lime
- 1 tbsp. extra-virgin olive oil
- 1/4 c. new cilantro leaves and delicate stems
- 1 garlic clove, minced
- 1/2 tsp. genuine salt
- FOR SERVING:
- 8 corn tortillas, warmed
- Salted red onions
- Cilantro leaves, for serving

DIRECTIONS:

1. Make smooth avocado sauce: consolidate all ingredients in a blender or food processor, and add 2/3 cups cold water. Mix until smooth.
2. Make lentil filling: In a large skillet over medium heat, heat oil. Add onion and cook until delicate, 6 minutes. Add garlic and cook until fragrant, brief more.
3. Add tomato paste and chipotle pepper, and cook, squashing pepper with a wooden spoon, until tomato paste has obscured marginally, 2 minutes. Add cumin and coriander and season with salt. Add lentils and ¼ cup cold water. Mix to consolidate, at that point cook, blending and pounding a portion of the lentils occasionally, until lentils are heated through and partially crushed, and no fluid remaining parts, around 5 minutes. Add more water a tablespoon at a time if skillet gets dry.

4. Collect tacos: fill every tortilla with a major spoonful of lentil blend, a sprinkle of sauce, red onions, and jalapeño.

2. Veggie Kabobs

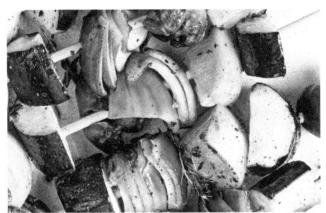

YIELDS:1 DOZEN PREP TIME:0 HOURS 30 MINS
TOTAL TIME:0 HOURS 45 MINS

INGREDIENTS:

- 2 medium zucchini, cut into 1" thick half-moons
- 1 (10-oz.) bundle infant bella mushrooms, cleaned and divided
- 1 medium red onion, cut into wedges
- 2 small lemons, cut into eighths
- 3 tbsp. extra-virgin olive oil
- 1 garlic clove, ground
- 1 tsp. newly chopped thyme, oregano, or rosemary
- Squeeze squashed red pepper drops
- Fit salt
- Newly ground black pepper

DIRECTIONS:

1. In the case of using wooden sticks, absorb water for 30 minutes. Preheat barbecue to medium-high heat.
2. String each stick with zucchini, mushrooms, onions, and lemon pieces, rotating each.
3. In a small bowl, whisk together oil, garlic, spices, and red pepper drops. Brush all over sticks, at that point season sticks with salt and pepper.
4. Barbecue, turning occasionally, until vegetables are delicate and somewhat scorched, 12 to 14 minutes. Serve hot.

3. Cannellini Beans With Herb Sauce

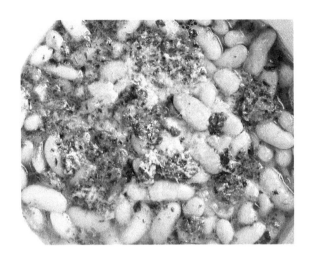

YIELDS: 6 SERVINGS PREP TIME: 0 HOURS 20 MINS TOTAL TIME: 0 HOURS 45 MINS

INGREDIENTS:

- 2 medium zucchini, cut into 1" thick half-moons
- 1 (10-oz.) bundle child bella mushrooms, cleaned and split
- 1 medium red onion, cut into wedges
- 2 small lemons, cut into eighths
- 3 tbsp. extra-virgin olive oil
- 1 garlic clove, ground
- 1 tsp. newly chopped thyme, oregano, or rosemary
- Squeeze squashed red pepper pieces
- Genuine salt
- Newly ground black pepper

DIRECTIONS:

1. In the case of using wooden sticks, absorb water for 30 minutes. Preheat barbecue to medium-high heat.
2. String each stick with zucchini, mushrooms, onions, and lemon pieces, substituting each.
3. In a small bowl, whisk together oil, garlic, spices, and red pepper pieces. Brush all over sticks, at that point season sticks with salt and pepper.
4. Barbecue, turning occasionally, until vegetables are delicate and somewhat roasted, 12 to 14 minutes. Serve hot.

4.　Perfect Bok Choy

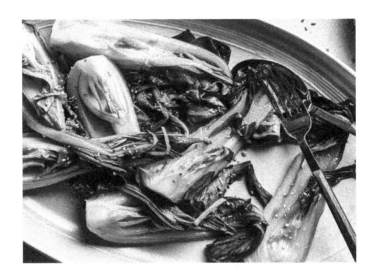

YIELDS:2 - 3 SERVINGS
PREP TIME:0 HOURS 5 MINS
TOTAL TIME:0 HOURS 10 MINS

INGREDIENTS

- 1 tbsp. vegetable oil
- 2 garlic cloves, minced
- 1" ginger, stripped and cut into slight matchsticks
- 1 lb. infant bok choy, cut in quarters with center unblemished
- 2 tsp. low-sodium soy sauce
- 1 tsp. toasted sesame oil, for serving (optional)
- 1/2 tsp. toasted sesame seeds, for serving (optional)

DIRECTIONS:

1. Heat vegetable oil in a large skillet over medium-high heat. Add garlic and ginger and cook until fragrant, 30 seconds.
2. Add bok choy, soy sauce, and 2 tablespoons water. Cover and cook 1 moment, at that point eliminate top and cook, blending occasionally, until centers are delicate and all fluid has dissipated. Move to a serving dish, shower with sesame oil and sprinkle with sesame seeds, if using.

5.   Rosemary Roasted Potatoes

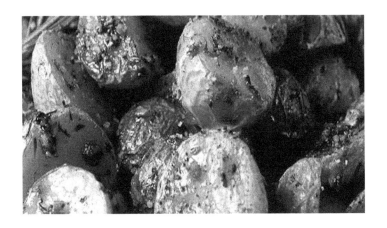

YIELDS:6 PREP TIME:0 HOURS 10 MINS TOTAL TIME:1 HOUR 10 MINS

INGREDIENTS:

- 2 lb. infant potatoes, divided or quartered assuming large
- 2 tbsp. extra-virgin olive oil
- 4 cloves garlic, minced
- 2 tbsp. newly chopped rosemary
- fit salt
- Newly ground black pepper
- New rosemary twigs, for serving

DIRECTIONS:

1. Preheat oven to 400º. Add potatoes to heating sheet. Throw with olive oil, garlic, and

rosemary and season liberally with salt and pepper.
2. Cook until fresh, mixing occasionally, 1 hour to 1 hour 15 minutes.
3. Add more rosemary branches for serving.

6. Kung Pao Brussels Sprouts

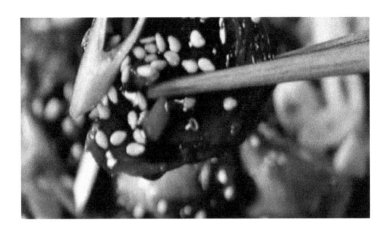

Yields:6 servings | prep time:0 hours 10 mins | total time:0 hours 35 mins

INGREDIENTS:

- 2 lb. Brussels sprouts, split
- 2 tbsp. extra-virgin olive oil
- Genuine salt
- Newly ground black pepper
- 1 tbsp. sesame oil
- 2 cloves garlic, minced
- 1 tbsp. cornstarch
- 1/2 c. low-sodium soy sauce
- 1/2 c. water
- 2 tsp. apple juice vinegar
- 1 tbsp. hoisin sauce
- 1 tbsp. stuffed brown sugar
- 2 tsp. garlic stew sauce
- Squeeze squashed red pepper chips

- Sesame seeds, for embellish
- Green onions, daintily cut, for embellish
- Chopped broiled peanuts, for decorate

DIRECTIONS:

1. Preheat oven to 425°. On a large rimmed heating sheet, throw Brussels with olive oil and season with salt and pepper.
2. Prepare until Brussels sprouts are delicate and somewhat fresh, around 20 minutes. Move Brussels fledglings to a large bowl (however keep the heating sheet nearby). Preheat oven.
3. In a small skillet over medium heat, heat sesame oil. Add garlic and cook, until fragrant, around 1 moment. Mix in cornstarch. Add soy sauce, water, apple juice vinegar, hoisin sauce, brown sugar, and garlic stew paste. Season with salt, pepper and red pepper pieces. Heat combination to the point of boiling, at that point diminish heat and stew until thickened, around 3 minutes.
4. Pour sauce over Brussels fledglings and throw to consolidate. Return Brussels fledglings to preparing sheet and sear until Brussels sprouts are coated and tacky.
5. Trimming with peanuts, sesame seeds, and green onions prior to serving.

7. Avocado Hummus

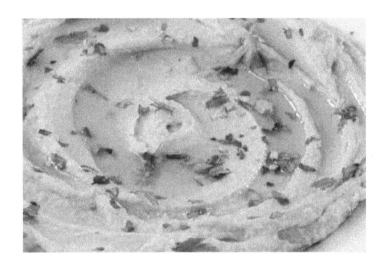

YIELDS:6 – 8 PREP TIME:0 HOURS **5** MINS
TOTAL TIME:0 HOURS **10** MINS

INGREDIENTS:

- 2 c. canned chickpeas
- 2 ready avocados, cored and stripped
- 1/3 c. tahini
- 1/4 c. lime juice
- 2 cloves garlic
- 3 tbsp. olive oil, in addition to additional for serving
- 1/4 tsp. cumin
- genuine salt
- 1 tbsp. Chopped cilantro, for embellish
- Red pepper pieces, for embellish

DIRECTIONS:

1. Consolidate chickpeas, avocados, tahini, lime juice, garlic, olive oil and cumin in the bowl of a food processor and season with salt. Mix until smooth.
2. Empty blend into serving bowl and trimming with cilantro and red pepper drops. Sprinkle with more olive oil whenever wanted and serve.

8. Vegan Lasagna

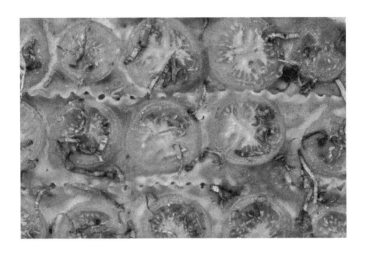

YIELDS:10 – 12 PREP TIME:0 HOURS 15 MINS
TOTAL TIME:1 HOUR 45 MINS

INGREDIENTS:

- FOR THE LASAGNA
- 1 box lasagna noodles
- 1 (14-oz) bundle firm tofu, depleted
- fit salt
- Newly ground black pepper
- 1 tbsp. olive oil
- 1 large onion, chopped
- 3 garlic cloves, minced
- 2 tsp. dried oregano, separated
- 1 (8-oz) bundle infant bella mushrooms, cut
- 2 (10-oz) bundles frozen spinach, defrosted and depleted of overabundance fluid
- FOR THE WHITE SAUCE
- 1/4 c. olive oil
- 1/4 c. all-purpose flour

- 2 1/2 c. almond milk (or other non-dairy milk)
- 2 tbsp. dietary yeast
- 1/2 tsp. garlic powder
- legitimate salt
- Newly ground black pepper
- 2 c. marinara
- 3 tomatoes, meagerly cut
- 1/4 c. meagerly cut basil, for decorate

DIRECTIONS;

1. Preheat oven to 350º. Heat a large pot of salted bubbling water to the point of boiling and cook lasagna noodles until still somewhat firm. Channel.
2. Enclose tofu by a spotless kitchen material or paper towels and spot on a large plate. Spot a container or weighty plate on top of tofu to press out however much fluid as could be expected. Let sit for in any event 30 minutes. When depleted, disintegrate with two forks and season with salt and pepper. Put away.
3. In a large skillet over medium heat, heat oil. Add onion and garlic and season with salt, pepper, and 1 tsp oregano. Add mushrooms and cook until mollified, 3 to 4 minutes. Mix in defrosted and depleted spinach until totally joined. Eliminate from heat and put away vegetables.
4. Crash skillet and get back to medium heat to make white sauce: Add olive oil and heat until gleaming yet not smoking. Add flour and race to consolidate. Cook until delicately golden and nutty, 1 to 2 minutes. Rush in nut milk until

smooth. Mix in wholesome yeast and garlic powder and season with salt and pepper. Bring to a stew and let cook until thickened, 8 to 10 minutes.

5. Construct lasagna: In a large preparing dish, spoon 1/4 c marinara into an even layer, at that point add a layer of noodles. Top with an even layer of vegetable blend, tofu, marinara, and white sauce. Rehash until all ingredients are utilized, finishing off with marinara. Add a solitary layer of tomato adjusts and season with salt, pepper and remaining oregano.

6. Prepare 35 to 40 minutes, until tomatoes are cooked and lasagna is heated through. Eliminate from oven and let cool marginally. Embellishment with basil and serve.

9.   Soused Red Cabbage

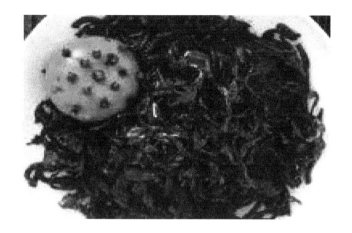

Prep:10 mins   Cook:5 mins   plus   2   hrs standingEasy Serves 4

Ingredients:

- 500g red cabbage (around 1/4 of a large head), center eliminated, meagerly cut
- 4 tbsp ocean salt
- ½ tsp dark peppercorns
- 2 cove leaves
- 1 rosemary branch
- 500ml juice vinegar
- 400g brilliant caster sugar
- 1 red onion , meagerly cut

Technique:

1. Combine as one the cabbage and salt in a large bowl. Put the peppercorns, cove and rosemary on a little piece of muslin material

and tie into a little zest sack. Smash the sack to deliver the flavors, at that point add to the red cabbage. Put away for 1 hr, giving it a mix after 30 mins.

2. Then, make the sousing fluid: bring the vinegar, sugar, onion and 50ml water to the bubble in a large container. Eliminate from the heat and leave to cool.

3. Eliminate the zest pack from the cabbage and drop it into the cooling fluid. Flush the cabbage well under running water to eliminate the salt, at that point press to dispose of the abundance water. Move the cabbage to a large cleaned Kilner container (see tip). Pour over the cooled sousing fluid, seal and put away to pickle for in any event 1 hr. Can be made as long as multi week ahead of time.

4. **Formula TIPS**

5. TO Sterilize YOUR JAR

6. Heat oven to 160C/140C fan/gas 3 and wash the container in hot sudsy water. While it's actually wet, stand it topsy turvy on a preparing plate and leave in the oven for 10 minutes.

10. Red Cabbage With Coriander Seed

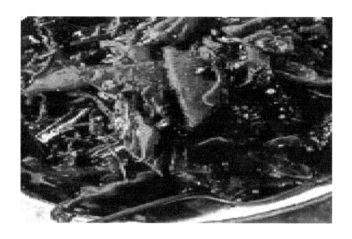

Prep:20 mins Cook:1 hr and 15 mins Easy Serves 6

Ingredients:

- 1 tbsp olive oil
- 1 red cabbage , around 900g, quartered, cored and shredded
- 1 onion , cut
- 1 garlic clove , chopped
- 1½ tbsp coriander seeds
- 2 narrows leaves
- 2 Granny Smith apples , stripped, cored and chopped
- 75ml great quality vegetarian white wine vinegar
- 50ml maple syrup

Technique:

1. Heat the oil in a large pan or goulash dish over a medium heat. Add the cabbage, onion, garlic, coriander seeds and narrows leaves, and cook, mixing at times, for 15 mins until the cabbage starts to wither.
2. Mix in the apple, vinegar and maple syrup and season well. Cover the skillet and cook delicately for 1 hr until the cabbage is delicate and superbly tacky and caramelized. Eliminate the straight leaves prior to eating. Can be made ahead of time and frozen or kept chilled for as long as two days. Go through any extras in our air pocket and squeak informal breakfast.

11. Savoy Cabbage With Shallots & Fennel Seeds

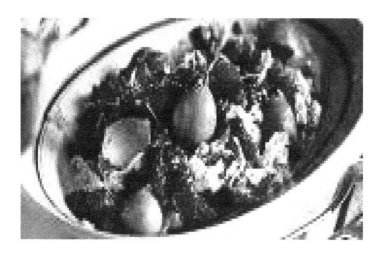

Prep:20 mins Cook:30 mins Easy Serves 8

Ingredients:

- 300g pack little shallots
- 2 tbsp olive oil
- 2 large garlic cloves , cut
- 1 tsp fennel seeds , delicately squashed
- 1 Savoy cabbage (external leaves disposed of) quartered, cored and shredded
- 150ml hot vegetable stock

Strategy:

1. Heat up the shallots in their skins for 10-15 mins until they are delicate yet hold their shape. Leave to cool at that point slip the skins from the shallots and divide them. Can be

several days ahead of time, at that point chilled.

2. Heat the oil in a large non-stick wok, and pan fried food the garlic, fennel seeds and shallots two or three mins until the shallots are brilliant. Eliminate from the dish.

3. Add the cabbage to the dish and pan fried food until it begins to shrivel somewhat, at that point pour in the stock, cover the wok and cook for 3 mins until simply delicate. Test to check whether the cabbage is done as you would prefer; on the off chance that not, cook somewhat more, add the shallot blend, heat through and serve.

12. Halloumi & Red Cabbage Steaks

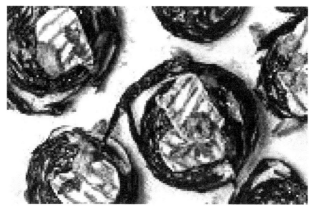

Prep:15 mins Cook:40 mins Easy Serves 4

Ingredients:

- 1 little red cabbage (about 900g/2lb), cut into 4 x 2cm/3/4in-thick 'steaks'
- 2 tbsp balsamic vinegar
- 2 tbsp olive oil
- 1 tsp fennel seeds
- 1 tbsp dull muscovado sugar
- 2 x 250g pockets prepared cooked quinoa
- juice 1 orange
- little pack level leaf parsley , chopped
- little pack dill , chopped
- 50g dried sharp cherry , generally chopped
- 250g pack halloumi , cut into 8 cuts

Strategy:

1. Heat oven to 200C/180C fan/gas 6. Line a preparing plate with heating material and put the cabbage steaks on top. Combine as one the balsamic, oil, fennel seeds and sugar, at that point season and spoon it over the cabbage. Cover the cabbage with foil and dish for 20 mins, at that point eliminate the foil and cook for a further 10 mins until softened.
2. Heat the quinoa adhering to pack directions, at that point mix through the squeezed orange, parsley, dill and cherries, and season with dark pepper. Fry the halloumi in a dry container on a medium heat for 2 mins each side until brilliant. To serve, place a spoonful of quinoa onto each cabbage steak and top with the halloumi.

13. Cabbage With Balsamic Vinegar

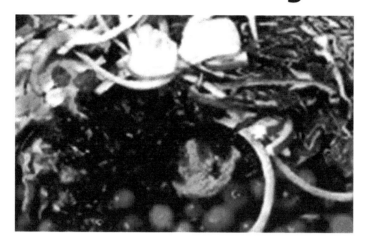

Prep:30 mins Cook:40 mins Easy Serves 8

Ingredients:

- 3 tbsp olive oil
- 2 large onions, split and daintily cut
- 1 tsp ground cloves
- 1 medium red cabbage, quartered, cored and daintily cut
- 200ml vegetable stock
- 3 tbsp balsamic vinegar
- 100g brown sugar
- 200g new or frozen cranberry

Strategy:

1. Heat the oil in a large container. Add the onions and fry, mixing occasionally, for around 10 mins, until they begin to caramelize. Mix in

the cloves, at that point add the cabbage and keep cooking, mixing all the more every now and again this time, until the cabbage begins to mollify.

2. Pour in the stock, add the vinegar and sugar, at that point cover and cook for 10 mins.
3. Mix in the cranberries and cook for 10 mins more. Cool and keep in the refrigerator for as long as 4 days, or freeze for multi month. Defrost in the ice chest short-term. Reheat until hot prior to serving.
4. **Formula TIPS**
5. Twofold DUTY
6. This preferences truly happy and incorporates new cranberries so you will not have to make a different cranberry sauce.
7. Works out in a good way For
8. Mustard, hotdog and apple tart
9. Juice broil turkey

14. Cabbage Steaks

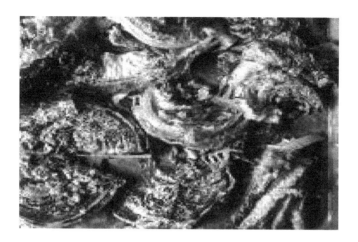

Prep:10 mins Cook:35 min Easy Serves 4 as a light meal or side

Ingredients:

- 1 firm, round cabbage
- 2 tbsp olive oil
- 1 tart, red-cleaned apple (we utilized Jazz)
- 1 tsp juice vinegar
- about 300g goat's cheddar (one with a skin from the cheddar counter) cut into four thick cuts (we utilized Soignon)
- 25g walnuts , generally broken
- a couple of thyme branches , leaves as it were
- great spot of cayenne pepper or hot smoked paprika
- 1 tbsp maple syrup

Technique:

1. Heat oven to 200C/180C fan/gas 6. Cut 4 x 2cm cuts from the center of the cabbage, slicing through the focal center and leaving it in. Brush done with virtually all the oil, season well, and spot on a preparing plate. Broil for 20 mins, turning cautiously using a fish cut or wide spatula part of the way through cooking.
2. While you stand by, meagerly cut the apple, leaving the skin on, at that point throw in a bowl with the vinegar and what's left of the oil.
3. Layer the apples on top of the cabbage steaks, broil for 5 mins more, at that point top every steak with a wheel of cheddar. Separation the nuts, thyme leaves and cayenne between each hill. Broil for a last 5 mins until the cheddar is beginning to dissolve and the walnuts are toasted. Shower with the maple syrup and consume straight.

15. Vegetarian Mushroom Gravy

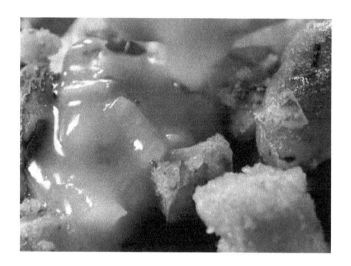

YIELDS:8 COOK TIME: 0 HOURS 10 MINS TOTAL TIME: 0 HOURS 15 MINS

INGREDIENTS:

- 2 tbsp. extra-virgin olive oil
- 1/2 Onion, finely chopped
- 4 oz. mushrooms, finely chopped
- legitimate salt
- Newly ground black pepper
- 1 tsp. chopped thyme
- 1 tsp. chopped sage
- 1 tsp. chopped rosemary
- 3 tbsp. all-purpose flour
- 3 c. vegetable stock

DIRECTIONS:

1. Heat olive oil in a small pot over medium heat. Add onion and sauté until delicate, 6 minutes. Mix in mushrooms and spices and season with salt and pepper. Cook until delicate, around 5 minutes more. Add flour and cook for 1 moment.
2. Pour in 2 cups of vegetable stock and rush to consolidate. Bring to stew and cook for 5-10 minutes, until the flavors have merged and the blend has thickened marginally. In the event that the combination is excessively thick, gradually add more vegetable stock.
3. Taste and season with more salt and pepper if necessary, at that point serve warm.

16. Prepared Oatmeal

Ingredients:

- 2 cups moved oats
- 1 tablespoon flaxseed dinner
- 1 teaspoon ground cinnamon
- 1/2 teaspoons without aluminum heating powder
- 2 1/4 cups rice milk
- 1 teaspoon unadulterated vanilla concentrate
- 1/2 cup chopped dried apricots for raisins
- 1/2 cup new blueberries
- Rice milk, for serving

Steps:

1. Preheat the oven to 350 degrees fahrenheit and softly oil a 8 x 8-inch heating dish.
2. In a large bowl, join all the ingredients and mix until very much consolidated.
3. Fill the prepared heating skillet and prepare uncovered for 30 minutes.
4. Cool marginally, at that point cut into 8 squares.
5. Serve warm, finished off with a little rice milk and additional cinnamon.

17. Banana-Ginger-Pear-Bowl

Ingredients:

- 1 banana
- 1 pear, stoned
- 1 date, stoned
- 3 tablespoons almonds
- 1 tablespoon flaxseeds
- 1 tablespoon hemp flour
- 1/2 tablespoon carob powder
- 1/2 tablespoon new ginger
- 250ml soy milk

Steps:

1. Cut the banana, pear, dates and almonds into pieces (size as you would prefer).
2. Put all the ingredients in a bowl-
3. Add the soy milk. Enjoy!

18. Breakfast Bowl

Ingredients:

- 1 banana
- 1 pear
- 1 date, stoned
- 3 tablespoons of almonds
- 1 tablespoons of flaxseeds
- 1/2 cup of millet chips
- 1/2 tablespoon of ground ginger
- 250ml soymilk

Steps:

1. Strip the banana.
2. Stone the pear.
3. Cut the banana, pear, almonds and the dates into minuscule pieces.
4. Put all the ingredients into a bowl.
5. Add the soymilk. Enjoy!

19. Waffles

Ingredients:

- 1 banana
- 1 cup entire wheat cake flour
- 1/4 teaspoon heating pop
- 1/2 teaspoon ocean salt
- 2 servings of Energ-G Egg Replacer with a large portion of the fluid called for on the bundle
- 1/4 cups almond milk or soy milk
- 1 teaspoon new lemon juice
- Nonstick cooking shower

Steps:

1. Freeze at that point defrost a banana and strip it. Squash the banana. Preheat a waffle iron.
2. In a medium bowl, join the flour, heating pop and salt. In another medium bowl, whip together the Ener-G Egg Replacer combination and add the pounded banana, almond or soy milk, and lemon juice. Add the wet ingredients to the dry ingredients and consolidate them thoroughly.
3. Give the waffle iron a speedy shower of nonstick cooking splash. Add a portion of the batter to your waffle iron (the sum relies upon the size of your iron, however ensure the iron is covered with a dainty layer of batter) and cook until golden brown, around 5 minutes.

4. Tenderly strip the waffle out of the iron with a flimsy cutting edge and rehash making waffles with the remainder of the batter.

20. Banana-Chocolate Pancakes

Ingredients:

- 2 stripped and pounded bananas
- 2 dried dates, stoned
- 20g amaranth
- 250ml chocolate hemp milk
- 250ml water
- 70g buckwheat flour
- 4 tablespoons of linseeds
- 4 tablespoons of hemp protein
- 3 tabespoons of carob powder
- 2 tablespoons of caca onibs

Steps:

1. Mix all these ingredients together.
2. Pour not very many coconut-oil (utilize an oil-shower) into a preparing skillet.
3. Empty the ingredients into the preparing dish until you have the correct size of the hotcake for you.
4. Heat for 5 minutes, go it to the opposite side and prepare for an additional 5 minutes.

21. Breakfast Wraps

Ingredients:

- 1 14-ounce bundle firm tofu, depleted
- 2 cloves garlic
- 1/2 cup diced onion
- 1 teaspoon ocean salt
- 1/4 teaspoon ground turmeric
- newly ground black pepper
- 4 entire grain tortillas
- 1/2 cup prepared salsa

Steps:

1. Channel the tofu and disintegrate it in a different bowl.
2. Heat a couple of tablespoons of water in a medium skillet over medium heat. Add the garlic, onion and a couple of portions of ocean salt. Cook for 5 minutes.
3. Spot the depleted and disintegrated tofu on top of the garlic and onion blend. Sprinkle with the turmeric, the excess ocean salt, and pepper to taste. Cover the skillet and cook for 3 minutes.
4. Spot one-fourth of the tofu blend in a tortilla. Add one-fourth of the salsa and wrap the tortilla gently around the filling. Rehash with the excess tortillas.

22. Banana Bread

Ingredients:

- 2 bananas, crushed well
- 1/3 cup blended black espresso
- 3 tablespoons chia seeds blended in with 6 tablespoons water and mixed well
- 1/2 cup olive oil
- 1/2 cup maple syrup
- 1 cup white flour and 1 cup wholemeal flour
- 2 tsp preparing powder
- 1/2 tsp salt
- 1 tsp every cinnamon and allspice

Steps:

1. Preheat the oven to 350°F and line a portion dish.
2. Beat together the delicate spread and sugar until cushioned, at that point add in the chia seed combination. In the case of using oil, simply combine all these ingredients as one.
3. Mix in the pounded bananas and espresso well.
4. Filter the flours, salt and raising specialists, at that point delicately overlay into the wet combination.
5. Heat in the oven for 30-40 minutes, until brown on top and a stick tells the truth.

23. Cinnamon-Quinoa-Breakfast

Ingredients:

- 1 cup soy milk
- 1 cup water
- 1 cup natural quinoa
- 2 cups new blackberries, natural liked
- 1/2 teaspoon ground cinnamon
- 1/3 cup chopped walnuts, toasted
- 4 teaspoons agave nectar

Steps:

1. Join the soy milk, water and quinoa in a medium pan. Heat to the point of boiling over high heat. Decrease heat to medium-low; cover and stew 15 minutes or until the greater part of the fluid is assimilated.
2. Mood killer heat; let stand covered 5 minutes. Mix in blackberries and cinnamon.
3. Move to four dishes and top with walnuts. Sprinkle 1 teaspoon agave nectar over each serving.

24. Japan-Like Lentil Breakfast

Ingredients:

- 2 tablespoons olive oil
- 1 medium leek, white and light green parts just, finely chopped
- 1 clove garlic, meagerly cut
- 1 tablespoon tomato paste
- 1 cup green lentils
- 2 tablespoons diminished sodium soy sauce
- Salt and newly ground black pepper

Steps:

1. Heat oil in a medium pot over medium heat. Add leek, garlic, and tomato paste and cook, mixing regularly, until fragrant and tomato paste starts to obscure.
2. Add lentils and 2½ cups water. Heat to the point of boiling; decrease heat, cover, and stew, mixing occasionally, until lentils are delicate.
3. Eliminate the skillet from heat and let it sit, covered for 10 minutes. Add soy sauce and season with salt and pepper.

25. Banana-Nut Oatmeal

Ingredients:

- 2 cups plain almond milk
- 2 completely matured large bananas (1/2 diced and 1/2 daintily cut transversely)
- 1/4 teaspoon unadulterated almond remove
- 1/4 teaspoon unadulterated vanilla concentrate
- 2 cups antiquated moved oats
- 2 tablespoons unsweetened cocoa powder
- 2 tablespoons agave nectar
- 1/3 cup toasted and chopped pecans
- Squeeze ground cinnamon
- 2 tablespoons semisweet chocolate chips
- touch of salt

Steps:

1. Bring the almond milk, 1 3/4 cups water, the diced bananas, almond and vanilla concentrates and touch of salt to a bubble in a large pot over high heat.
2. Mix in the oats, cocoa powder and 1 tablespoon of the agave nectar and diminish the heat to medium. Cook, blending every now and again, until the oats are completely cooked to wanted consistency, 6 to 7 minutes.
3. Move to 4 dishes, top with the cut bananas, pecans, the excess 1 tablespoon agave nectar, cinnamon and chocolate chips and serve.

26. Almond-Flaxseed-Burger

Ingredients:

- 2 garlic cloves
- 1 cup of almonds
- 6 tablespoons of flaxseeds
- 2 tablespoons of apple juice vinegar
- 2 tablespoons of coconut oil

Steps:

1. Mix all the ingredients together.
2. Structure two burger patties. You can eat these vegan-meat-patties crude or put some coconut oil on them and put them into a preparing skillet at medium heat.
3. Cook until they're golden.
4. Add them to two entire grain slices of bread.
5. Add a few vegetables for additional taste.

27. Chickpeas-Curry-Pizza

Ingredients:

- 230g of grounded sunflower seeds
- 180g of cooked chickpeas
- 60ml of coconut oil
- 1 tablespoon of cloves
- 1 tablespoon of curry powder
- 1/2 tablespoon of curcuma

Fixings:

- 1/2 medium measured sweet potato
- 1/2 onion, cut
- 1/2 piece of broccoli (floweret)
- 1/2 piece of cauliflower (floweret)

Steps:

1. Preheat the oven to 300 degrees fahrenheit.
2. Mix all the ingredients for the hull together.
3. Mix it until it structures bumps.
4. Put some coconut-fat on the heating plate.
5. Convey the mixed mass equally on the heating plate.
6. Add the garnishes.
7. Prepare for aprroximately 45 minutes in the oven. Preparing time can be changed, as indicated by your preferences.

28. Amaranth-Hemp Seeds-Salad

Ingredients:

- 1 Nori leaf, chopped
- 4 modest bunch of blended plates of mixed greens
- 10g of amaranth
- 1 modest bunch of sugar snaps
- 2 tablespoons of hemp seeds

Steps:

1. Put all the ingredients in a bowl.
2. Add some dressing, I suggest an italian dressing.
3. Ensure you utilize just a smidgen of oil.

29. Sweet Potato Burritos

Ingredients:

- 2 cups stripped and cut sweet potatoes
- 1 cup frozen corn portions
- 1 15-ounce can low-sodium black beans, depleted and washed
- 1 teaspoon daintily cut green onion
- 1 tablespoon new lime juice
- 1 tablespoon bean stew powder
- ocean salt and newly ground black pepper
- 4 8-inch entire wheat tortillas, warmed
- 1 cup prepared salsa
- 2 cups shredded lettuce

Steps:

1. Spot the sweet potatoes in a medium pot and add water to come an inch up the sides. Spot over medium-high heat and heat to the point of boiling; cook for 5 minutes.
2. Add the corn and cook 1 more moment.
3. Channel and move to a large bowl. Add the black beans, green onion, lime juice and stew powder; season with salt and pepper to taste.
4. Split the filling between the tortillas, top with the salsa and lettuce, move them up, and serve.

30. Spaghetti With White Bean Marinara Sauce

Ingredients:

- 10 ounces uncooked entire grain spaghetti
- 1 24-ounce jar without fat spaghetti sauce
- 1 15-ounce can low-sodium cannellini beans, depleted and washed

Steps:

1. Cook the spaghetti as per the bundle directions; channel.
2. In the interim, in a medium pot, join the spaghetti sauce and beans, cover, and warm over low heat.
3. Serve the spaghetti finished off with the marinara-bean blend.

31. Prepared Ziti

Ingredients:

- 1/2 teaspoon olive oil
- 8 ounces uncooked entire grain ziti or penne pasta
- 10.5 ounces firm low-fat tofu, depleted
- 2 tablespoons entire wheat cake flour
- 1 teaspoon garlic powder
- 1 teaspoon onion powder
- 1 teaspoon dried basil
- 1/2 teaspoon dried oregano
- 1/2 teaspoon ocean salt
- 1 24-ounce jar without fat spaghetti sauce

Steps:

1. Preheat the oven to 375°F and lube a 2 1/2-quart meal dish with the oil.
2. Cook the pasta as indicated by the bundle directions to still somewhat firm.
3. Disintegrate the depleted tofu into a bowl and add the flour, garlic powder, onion powder, basil, oregano and salt. Blend well.
4. Delicately overlap in the cooked pasta, spaghetti sauce, and any optional ingredients.
5. Spoon the pasta-tofu combination into the prepared goulash dish and heat for 25 minutes or until firm and daintily golden on top. Serve hot with a new nursery salad.

32. Gnocchi With Basil And Sun-Dried Tomatoes

Ingredients:

- 4 to 6 basil leaves, cut into strips
- 1/2 cups without dairy whoel wheat gnocchi
- 10 to 12 sun-dried tomatoes
- 1 teaspoon broke black pepper

Steps:

1. Lay the basil leaves on top of each other, move them up, and cut them into strips.
2. Heat a medium pot of water to the point of boiling. Add the gnocchi and mix; cook until the gnocchi skim.
3. Eliminate them really the highest point of the water and channel.
4. Move to a serving bowl and throw the gnocchi with the basil strips, sun-dried tomatoes, and pepper and serve.

33. Prepared Veggie Falafel

Ingredients:

- 1 15-ounce can low-sodium garbanzo beans, depleted and washed
- 2 tablespoons minced onion
- 1 clove garlic, minced
- 1 tablespoon minced new parsley
- 1/4 cup shredded carrot
- 1 tablespoon new lemon juice
- 2 tablespoons entire wheat baked good flour
- 1 teaspoon ground coriander seeds
- 1 teaspoon ground cumin
- 1/4 cup cooked green peas
- Ocean salt and newly ground black pepper

Steps:

1. Preheat the oven to 350°F and gently oil a heating sheet.
2. Spot the garbanzo beans, onion, garlic, parsley, carrot, lemon juice, flour, coriander, and cumin in a food processor and interaction until genuinely smooth. Move the combination to a medium bowl and mix in the peas. Season with salt and pepper to taste.

   Structure the combination into 8 patties and spot them on the prepared heating sheet. Heat for 15 minutes, at that point cautiously turn the patties over and prepare for 15 additional minutes. Serve 2 patties stuffed inside an entire wheat pita pocket.

3. Top with a little hummus, shredded lettuce and diced onion and tomato. The patties additionally are extraordinary presented with couscous and a plate of mixed greens.

34. Grilled Eggplant Niçoise

Ingredients:

- 4 cloves garlic
- 1 large eggplant, cut into thick chunks
- Juice of 4 lemons
- 1/4 teaspoon broke black pepper
- 1 tablespoon dried lavender
- 1/2 teaspoon saffron
- 4 large cuts French bread, toasted
- 1 small fennel bulb, cut
- 2 tomatoes, cut
- 1/4 cup cut pitted Niçcoise olives or green olives

Steps:

1. Crush the garlic and rub every piece of eggplant with the garlic. Spot the eggplant in a shallow bowl and pour the lemon juice over it.
2. Add sufficient water to lower the eggplant. Allow the eggplant to marinate for in any event 60 minutes, at that point channel and spot it in a shallow dish.
3. Add the garlic, pepper, lavender, and saffron and let it sit for around 60 minutes.
4. Spot the eggplant straightforwardly on a barbecue over medium heat and cook until it is delicate on the two sides yet not roasted.
5. Spot a grilled section of eggplant on a cut of bread and top a few cuts of fennel and

tomatoes and around 1 tablespoon cut olives. This sandwich is served open confronted.

35. Tofu Scramble

Ingredients:

- 1 teaspoon olive oil
- ¼ cup onions, chopped
- 1 cup red and green chime peppers, chopped
- 1 cup spinach
- 12-14 ounces tofu, disintegrated
- Salt and pepper, to taste

Steps:

1. Heat oil in a skillet, add onions and peppers. Sauté until vegetables are mellowed.
2. Add spinach, disintegrated tofu, salt and pepper.
3. Cook for a couple of moments on medium heat and serve.
4. Sides
5. The dishes enhancing your full suppers – or dishes that can be a full dinner. In case you're a lethargic cook like me.

36. Toasted Brown Rice

Cooking mysterious: Toast rice first and afterward cook it like pasta.

Ingredients:

- 1 cup short-grain brown rice
- 3 cups water

Steps:

1. In a pan, wash the rice momentarily with water, at that point pour off as a large part of the water as possible. You are presently left with soggy rice.
2. Spot the container over high heat and mix the rice until dry, 1 to 2 minutes. Add the water, heat to the point of boiling, at that point decrease the heat and stew for around 40 minutes, until the rice is cooked – yet crunchy. Channel off any excess water.
3. Additional Step: To serve, top with sunflower or flaxseeds for that extra crunchiness.

37. Red Rice

Ingredients:

- 1/2 yellow onion, chopped
- 4 tomatillos, chopped
- 1/4 cups water
- 1 teaspoon white vinegar
- 1/2 teaspoon ocean salt
- 1 cup brown rice

Steps:

1. Heat a medium pan over medium heat; add the onion and cook until it is clear, around 3 to 4 minutes, blending at regular intervals or somewhere in the vicinity.
2. Add the tomatoes, water, vinegar, and salt and bring to a stew. Add the rice and get back to a stew.
3. Cover, and decrease the heat to low, and cook for around 25 minutes.

38. Mint Couscous

Ingredients:

- 3/4 cup hot mint tea
- 3/4 cup uncooked couscous
- 4 to 5 dried apricots
- 8 to 10 pitted dried black olives or pitted entire kalamata olives
- 1 tablespoon chile paste, ideally harissa sauce
- 1/3 cup cooked chickpeas, depleted and washed

Steps:

1. Join the hot tea and couscous in a medium bowl.
2. As the couscous retains the fluid, gradually cushion it with a fork.
3. Add the excess ingredients, mix together and serve.

39. Banana Ice Cream

Ingredients:

- Ready Bananas

Steps:

1. Strip and cut the bananas, place them in a compartment and freeze them for 60 minutes.
2. Eliminate the frozen bananas from the cooler and let them defrost a little at room temperature.
3. Spot the bananas in a food processor and cycle until smooth and velvety, as delicate serve frozen yogurt.
4. You can shift the recipe by adding a little cinnamon, vanilla or cocoa powder.

40. Organic Product Pops

Ingredients:

- Around 3 cups unsweetened organic product juice of your decision, like grape, pomegranate or squeezed orange (press at home and utilize the mash for more medical advantages)

Steps:

1. Fill an ice pop shape (set of 6) with the juice, put a wooden stick in there.
2. Allow it to freeze several hours.
3. To eliminate a frozen fly from the shape, run momentarily under warm water.

41. Blueberry Mini Muffin

Ingredients:

- 2 cup entire wheat spelt flour
- 2 tsp heating powder
- ½ tsp salt
- 2 cup natural blueberries
- ½ cup vegetable oil
- ½ cup soy milk
- ½ cup 100% maple syrup
- ¼ cup agave nectar

Steps:

1. Preheat oven to 375°F and fix a little cupcake tin with paper cups.
2. Combine wet ingredients as one in large bowl, at that point mix in dry ingredients, trailed by the blueberries.
3. Using small spoons, split the batter between the cups so they're nearly filled to the top.
4. Prepare until biscuits are golden brown, for around 20 minutes.

42. Vanilla Berry Sorbet

Ingredients:

- 2 cups new or frozen raspberries or strawberries
- 1 teaspoon of unadulterated vanilla concentrate
- 1/4 cup date sugar

Steps:

1. In a blender, join all the ingredients and mix until smooth.
2. Change the sweetness with the date sugar add up to taste if necessary.
3. Fill a cooler compartment, cover and freeze a few hours.
4. To serve, eliminate the sorbet from cooler and let remain at room temperature until sufficiently delicate to scoop out.

43. Peanut Butter Chocolate Ice Cream

Ingredients:

- 2 cut and frozen bananas
- 2 Tbsp common peanut butter
- 3 Tbsp crude cacao nibs
- Squeeze ocean salt
- Shower of agave (or maple syrup), optional

Steps:

1. Spot frozen banana cuts in a food processor and run the machine until it takes after a morsel like consistency.
2. Add peanut butter, cacao nibs, ocean salt and agave, and marvel somewhat more until you get a delicate serve frozen yogurt consistency.

44. Coconut Cashew Rice Pudding

Ingredients:

- 1 cup cashew milk
- 1 cup coconut milk
- ¼ cup Arborio rice
- 2 tsp stevia
- 2 tsp finely ground lime zing
- 1 tsp vanilla concentrate
- new berries, coconut, and additionally toasted cashews for decorate

Steps:

1. Spot the cashew milk, coconut milk, rice, sugar and lime zing in a medium saucepot and whisk while bringing it up to a stew over medium heat. Cover freely and keep on stewing delicately, blending regularly, until the rice is delicate, around 25 minutes. Eliminate the pot from the heat and mix in the vanilla. Cool the pudding to room temperature and afterward chill prior to serving.
2. Serve the pudding embellished with new berries, coconut shavings or potentially toasted cashews.

45. Prepared Fruit Compote

Ingredients:

- 4 cups cut peaches
- 1 cup blueberries
- 1/2 cup red raspberries
- 5 tablespoons maple syrup
- 1/2 teaspoon ground cinnamon
- 1/4 teaspoon ground allspice
- 1/4 teaspoon ground ginger
- 1/4 teaspoon ground cloves

Steps:

1. Preheat the oven to 350°F
2. Consolidate all the ingredients in a large bowl and blend delicately.
3. Empty the natural product into a 2-quart heating dish, cover and prepare for 30 minutes or until the organic product is delicate. Serve warm.

46. Frosted Watermelon And White Peach

Ingredients:

- 2 cups pureed white peaches
- 2 cups pureed watermelon
- 1/2 cup agave nectar
- Optional: Leavces from 1 small twig of mint, ideally lemon mint

Steps:

1. Eliminate the stems and pits from the peaches. Eliminate the seeds and skin from the watermelon. P
2. ribbon the peaches in the blender and puree them, at that point add the watermelon to the blender and puree once more. Add the agave nectar and mix to join.
3. Spot the pureed blend in a shallow metal or glass bowl and leave it in the cooler until it frosts over. With a large metal spoon, scratch the frozen combination to make a shaved ice treat.

47. Fruity Couscous Cake

Ingredients:

- 4 cups squeezed apple
- 1 teaspoon unadulterated vanilla concentrate
- spot of ocean salt
- 2 cups uncooked couscous
- 2 cups blueberries
- 1/2 cup all-organic product jam
- 1/2 cups new product of your decision

Steps:

1. Join the squeezed apple, vanilla and salt in a medium pot, bring to the bubble and add the couscous. Mix, cover and lessen the heat to low; stew for around 2 minutes. Mood killer the heat and put away, covered, for 5 to 10 minutes.
2. Tenderly crease the blueberries into the cooked couscous. Flush yet don't dry a 9 1/2 inch tart container. Empty the couscous blend into it and smooth the top with a spatula. Spot the cake in the cooler and chill for at any rate 2 hours or until firm.
3. Spread the jam over the cake and orchestrate the new organic product in a lovely example over the top.

48. Lemon Rice

Ingredients:

- Juice of 1 lemon
- 3/4 cup sweetened almond milk
- 1/2 teaspoon ground cinnamon
- 2 tablespoons currants
- 1/4 cup short-grain brown rice
- Zing of 1 lemon

Steps:

1. Zing a lemon and afterward squeeze it. Join the almond milk, lemon juice, cinnamon and currants in a medium pot and heat everything to the point of boiling.
2. Mix in the rice. Take the fluid back to bubble, cover the pot, diminish the heat to low and cook until the rice is delicate, around 20 minutes. There should in any case be a touch of fluid left in the pot.
3. Split the rice between serving bowls and top with the lemon zing.
4. Refreshments and Smoothies
5. Tip for making a smoothie: Remember to begin with the slowest speed at the blender and gradually amp it up. In any case the ingredients will not mix together as great as they ought to.

49. Chocolate-Hemp Milk

Ingredients:

- 875ml of water
- 135g of hemp seeds
- 2 tablespoons of carob powder
- 2 tablespoons of date sugar

Steps:

1. Mix all the ingredients together in a blender. Basic.
2. 35. In a hurry Smoothie

Ingredients:

- 1 ready banana
- 2 cups frozen organic product (I lean toward raspberries)
- 1 cup nondairy milk (I incline toward soy)

Steps:

1. Join all the ingredients in a blender. Mix for around 2 minutes.

50. Crunchy Smoothie

Ingredients:

- 3/4 cup Breakfast Smoothie (see #2 Smoothie)
- 1/4 cup toasted dried oats
- New berries

Steps:

1. Layer 1/4 cup of the smoothie at the lower part of a glass.
2. Add a 2-tablespoon layer of oats next.
3. Followed by another 1/4 cup of smoothie, at that point the last 2 tablespoons oats.
4. Polish it off with the last 1/4 cup of smoothie.
5. Top with new berries. Crunchy and delicious.

51. Blueberry-Antioxidant-Smoothie

Ingredients:

- 1 ready banana
- 3 cups of cold water
- 1 cup of blueberries
- 1 tablespoon of flaxseeds
- 1 tablespoon of agave syrup/stevia sweetener
- 1 tablespoon of crushed rooibos

Steps:

1. Consolidate all the ingredients in a blender.

Conclusion

I would like to thank you for choosing this book. It contains recipes which are easy to prepare and are according to vegan diet. Vegan food varieties will in general be lower in calories than creature determined ones, making it simpler to accomplish a sound body weight without actively focusing on cutting calories. Must give these a try and enjoy along with your family members.

CPSIA information can be obtained
at www.ICGtesting.com
Printed in the USA
LVHW050351210621
690717LV00009B/528